THE ARTHRITIS DIET

How to Eat to Relieve Your Pain

James Amir

CONTENTS

THE ARTHRITIS DIET

How to Eat to Relieve your Pain

INTRODUCTION

I want to thank you and congratulate you for downloading the book, "The Arthritis Diet – How to Eat to Relieve your Pain". This book contains proven steps and strategies on how to adapt a healthy diet that can aid with arthritis treatment and pain relief.

Arthritis can feel impossible to overcome, especially when most treatments for arthritis are only mildly effective. But many people have found relief through improved diet and lifestyle.

Through applying the tips in this book, I can guarantee you that you will be able to improve your symptoms. The diet provided in this book is proven by science and experience.

This book explains the last 30 years of research on arthritis and nutrition. However, feel free to simply skip to the getting started page and begin to take action at any time. You do not have to understand how the diet works to benefit from this book, although having an understanding will increase your desire to follow the diet.

Thanks again for downloading this book, I hope you enjoy it!

James Amir

CHAPTER 1: ARTHRITIS OVERVIEW - CAUSES AND SYMPTOMS

Arthritis is one of the most common and painful conditions suffered by more than 27 million people in the United States alone. Mostly experienced by seniors, arthritis can deeply affect the quality of life of its sufferers, causing them to struggle when performing even the simplest tasks as bending to pick up something off the floor.

Arthritis Definition And Causes

In simple terms, arthritis is the inflammation of the joints caused by one or more factors, depending on the nature of the condition. There are currently several types of arthritis known today, the most common one being osteoarthritis, mostly suffered by people in their 50s or more.

Certain situations can also put you at greater risk of arthritis including genetics, obesity, certain jobs that involve repetitive physical activity, injury, infections, autoimmune disease, and others. As the title suggests, this book will guide you through the proper care and treatment of arthritis using the right diet. Prior to doing that however, it's important that you first find out exactly what the condition entails and what type you have. From there, you can address the condition's triggers and causes to ensure a more effective and safe way of treating the condition.

Types of Arthritis Medical professionals have identified several other types of joint inflammation that may hit seniors, children, men, and women in all walks of life. Here's a rundown of the different types today:

Osteoarthritis – The cartilage – which covers the end of two bones to prevent them from rubbing on each other – starts to wear down overtime. When this happens, the bones eventually touch each other, causing pain. This is one of the most common forms of arthritis today and is usually triggered by long-term use of the bones and joints. If your job entails repetitive motion (lifting, bending), then chances are your arthritis is caused by the cartilage's wear and tear.

Rheumatoid arthritis – this is the most common type of arthritis known today, usually affecting one or more joints. It is actually defined as an autoimmune disease which basically means that the body is launching an attack on the joints, therefore causing pain. Unlike osteoarthritis, rheumatoid arthritis often occurs on both sides of the body. For example, if the left knee is suffering from the pain, the right knee will soon follow. The reason for rheumatoid arthritis is not exactly known.

Psoriatic Arthritis – this type of arthritis is basically a skin condition that extends to the joints. Stemming from psoriasis, the condition is characterized by red, puffy, and scaly patches of skin that is usually present along the knees and elbows. Psoriatic arthritis is not curable but treatable and may appear at any time when a person reaches 30 years old. Note though that the skin condition usually occurs first followed by the arthritic symptoms. Hence, if you are currently suffering from psoriasis now or have a family history of the case, there's a risk of having this disease as you get older.

Gout – although the word "arthritis" is not attached to it, gout is also considered a form of joint inflammation. The condition is caused by an abundance of uric acid in the body, leading to crystals that eventually trigger the pain in the joints. Typically experienced by men, gout is often felt along the big toe and the thumb.

Arthritis Diagnosis And Treatment

Diagnosis of arthritis is the first step towards proper treatment. Typically, the condition is diagnosed through physical examination in which the doctor would ask for your symptoms. Lab tests may also be performed to detect the presence of any chemicals or minerals that may be causing joint pain. Note that self-diagnosis is never a good idea, especially since there are several types of arthritis.

Once diagnosis has been made and your arthritis has been properly labeled within the right type, the next step is treatment. There are several ways to treat arthritis:

- Medication, mostly for pain management. Some pills are made to help with the protection of the cartilage, but this is not always the case.

- Surgery is a last resort, often used when the pain or joints are well-past medicinal treatment.

- Lifestyle changes such as exercise and diet are also common treatments prescribed by doctors. They are often taken together with medication, depending on the severity of the condition.

As already mentioned, this eBook will focus on the third arthritis treatment.

CHAPTER 2: DIET AND ARTHRITIS

There have been two diets studied extensively by researchers for treating arthritis – vegetarian and vegan diets and the Mediterranean diet. Both have been shown to reduce the levels of pain and joint swelling from arthritis.

Vegetarian And Vegan Diets

Vegetarian diets aim to exclude all meat (red meat, poultry, seafood) from the diet. Vegan diets exclude all animal products, including honey, eggs, and dairy from the diet. By doing so they tend to become what some doctors have coined, a 'whole-foods plant based (WFPB) diet' – the bulk of the diet is formed around the consumption of fruit and starch for carbohydrates, and nuts, legumes, seeds, and grains for protein.

There is over 30 years of research on WFPB diets and arthritis. Starting in 1979, arthritis researcher Lars Skoldstam and his team found that placing people with rheumatoid arthritis on a vegetable juice and fruit juice diet resulted in a remarkable reduction of pain and swelling in them after just 7 to 10 days [1]. In 1983 Skoldstam confirmed his findings by placing 19 rheumatoid arthritis patients on a WFPB vegan diet for 3 months. He noted that 11 of them showed improvement [2].

Some of the most compelling evidence for the WFPB diet's ability to treat rheumatoid arthritis comes from a study lead by arthritis researcher Jen Kjeldsen-Kragh [3]. In the study Jen Kjeldsen-Kragh and his team began by allocating 27 rheumatoid arthritis sufferers to an experiment group and 26 to a control group. The participants in the experiment group were sent off to a health farm for 4 weeks. At the farm they fasted for close to a week and were then fed a WFPB vegan diet, rich in potatoes, fruit, and vegetables. Conversely, the control group was sent to a convalescent home for 4 weeks where, instead of being fed a WFPB vegan diet, they followed an ordinary omnivourous diet- rich in meat and poultry.

In addition the basic diet the participants in the experiment group implemented a basic rotation diet (more on this later), to help identify any individual food sensitivities that exasperated their arthritis. Every second day they introduced a new food item – If they noticed increased pain, stiffness, or joint swelling within 1-2 days, the food was omitted from the diet for at least 7 days before being reintroduced. If symptoms flared up again, the food item was excluded from the diet permanently.

Once the participants from both groups left the farm, the experiment group continued their WFPB vegan diet for another 3.5 months, and then followed a WFPB lacto-vegetarian diet, adding in milk products for protein, for another 8.5 months. The control group remained on their omnivorous diet. After 13 months in total on the diet, the results showed that the experiment group experienced an improvement in reported well-being, stronger grip strength, and less number of tender joints!

In 1990's Dr John McDougal began to popularize the 'McDougal diet' - a very low fat WFPB vegan diet for treating arthritis. Dr McDougal had many successes with the diet, ranging from people putting their rheumatoid arthritis to degenerative arthritis disease in remission.

In 2002 Dr McDougal decided it was time to put his diet to the test in a clinical study [4]. McDougal put 24 patients with moderate to severe rheumatoid arthritis on his very low fat WFPB vegan diet for four-weeks. The diet was validated - all rheumatoid symptomatology decreased significantly, except for morning stiffness, and c-reactive protein (a measure of inflammation) decreased by 16%.

Finally, in 2015 arthritis researcher Chelsea Clinton and her team put 19 osteoarthritis sufferers on a WFPB vegan diet and compared them to 18 patients on a standard western omnivorous diet [5]. The researchers found significant reduction in pain compared to an ordinary omnivorous diet, with significant pain reduction seen as early as two weeks after initiation of dietary modification.

Mediterranean Diet

The Mediterranean diet is based on the traditional eating patterns of southern Italy, Greece and Spain. The core of the diet is based on the consumption of olive oil, legumes, fruits and vegetables, with moderate consumption of fish and dairy products. The diet is low on meat products.

Although the Mediterranean diet does not have the same amount of research behind it as a WFPB, a key study in 2003 validated the diet's ability to treat rheumatoid arthritis [6]. In the study a total of 56 patients with rheumatoid arthritis were enrolled – 29 were assigned to eat a Mediterranean style diet and 27 were assigned to eat a standard American diet for 12 weeks. After 12 weeks, the Mediterranean dieters experienced increased vitality, increased quality of life, and decreased rheumatoid arthritis disease activity.

How The Diets Work

So if both of these diets work, should you follow the WFPB diet or Mediterranean diet? Before making that decision it is important to understand why both diets are successful at treating arthritis.

Arachidonic Acid Metabolism Inhibition

The main reason why these diets work is because they greatly reduce intake of meat, which changes the body's fatty acid profile. In particular, diets low on meat are low in one fatty acid called arachidonic acid. Arachidonic acid is what's known as a precursor to pro-inflammatory prostaglandins – it is needed to create the molecules which cause pain in the body.

Reducing arachidonic acid intake has a similar effect to taking nonsteroidal anti-inflammatory drugs (NSAIDS). This is because NSAIDs work to reduce pain by inhibiting the COX-2 Enzyme. The COX-2 enzyme converts arachidonic acid to inflammatory prostaglandins. So by reducing your intake of arachidonic acid by eating the WFPB or Mediterranean diet, you are achieving pain reduction in a similar way to taking NSAIDs.

The effect of decreasing arachidonic acid consumption in arthritis patients can achieve profound results. A study in 1981 found that a fat-free diet resulted in complete remission in 6 patients with rheumatoid arthritis [7]. Although a fat free diet is unsustainable, because a small amount of fat is essential, the researchers concluded, "...dietary fats in amounts normally eaten in the American diet cause the inflammatory joint changes seen in rheumatoid arthritis."

Mediterranean dieters have higher serum levels of omega-3 fats than standard American diet eaters. Omega 3 fats are abundant in the foods the Mediterranean diet is centered on; fish, legumes, vegetables and soy. The metabolism of omega 3 fats produces anti-inflammatory prostaglandins. These prostaglandins contribute to a reduction in pain symptoms.

The Mediterranean diet also includes olive oil in the diet. Olive oil, like omega-3, inhibits inflammation. This is because of the compound oleocanthal in olive oil that inhibits the production

of COX-2 enzymes (the precursors to inflammatory prostaglandins).

CHAPTER 3: GETTING STARTED AND THE ROTATION DIET

As you have seen, WFPB diets and the Mediterranean diet are two scientifically proven diets to treat arthritis. People who stick to these diets see improvements in their levels of pain and joint swelling. These diets work because they are low in overall fat and inhibit the metabolism of the inflammatory prostaglandin fatty acid precursor arachidonic acid.

The best anti-arthritis diet is a hybrid; one that is low fat and based around plant foods – fruits, vegetables, starches, grains – like the WFPB. It is also one that obtains small amounts of anti-inflammatory fats such as omega 3 fats from fish and olive oil like the Mediterranean diet. High fat animal products like beef, poultry, eggs, and full-fat dairy should be avoided, only consumed on occasion. High fat foods like nuts and added oils should also be avoided.

However, it's important to appreciate that everyone is individual – some specific foods can trigger arthritic flares for one person but not another. This is because every time you eat a small amount of protein molecules from food can get into the bloodstream. The body makes antibodies to these proteins from foods that are not solely specific to them, but also interact with similar human proteins. This is known as molecular mimicry. This causes the body to attack itself (auto-immune disease) causing inflammation seen in rheumatoid and psosric arthritis.

For example, wheat, cereals, grains and low fat milk may be part of an anti-arthritis diet for some, but others might have to avoid them as they have been reported to trigger arthritis symptoms. The proteins in these foods are similar to proteins found in the body and set-off an auto-immune attack which causes inflammation in the joints. For example, in 1992, arthritis researcher Dr. Sheignalet reported on forty-six adults with rheumatoid arthritis who removed cereal and dairy products from their diet. 36 patients (78%) responded favorably with 17 clearly improved, and 19 in complete remission for one to five years. Medication was stopped in eight of those nine-teen with no relapse [8.]

Therefore, it's important to begin with a rotation diet first to see if you have any individual food triggers, instead of just starting on an anti-arthritis diet. For 14 days, your diet should consist of only the following three foods least likely to cause any problems in your body;

Sweet Potato

Non citrus fruits

Green and yellow vegetables

For the first two days eat only those foods and drink water – you should notice a marked improvement in your arthritis symptoms. Then, in addition to the basic safe foods diet, you are to introduce a new food item from the following list every second day:

Corn (Day 2)

Rice (Day 4)

Beans (Day 6)

Citris fruits (Day 8)

Night shades (Day 10)

Wheat (Day 12)

Low-fat Dairy (Day 14)

If you notice increased pain, stiffness, or joint swelling within 2–48 h, omit the food from the diet for at least 7 days before reintroducing it. If symptoms are exacerbated again, the food item is one of your individual triggers and should be avoided.

CHAPTER 4: SUPPLEMENTS

I n addition to an arthritis healthy diet, you can use supplements to further reduce inflammation and improve symptoms. Four proven supplements are vitamin D, ginger, curcumin, and gelatin.

Vitamin D

Vitamin D, also known as the sunshine vitamin, isn't actually a vitamin. It's actually a natural steroid-hormone your body produces when your skin comes into contact with ultraviolet b (UVB) from sunlight. However, this essential vitamin is also commonly found in some foods such as oily fish (salmon, mackerel) and is mainly used to fortify milk, cereal, and juice.

Vitamin D helps arthritis because of its beneficial effect on the immune system. In rheumatoid arthritis and psoriatic arthritis the immune system is overactive and out of balance, which causes the system to go awry and misreads signals. As a result, our defenses do not recognize our own body at work, and begin "attacking" cells. In Rheumatoid arthritis this leads to an inflammation of the joints. In psoriatic arthritis this leads to inflammation of the skin. Vitamin D re-balances the immune system. When arthritis sufferers increase their levels from deficient to healthy levels their immune systems calm down and joint pain decreases.

Vitamin D is most easily obtained from exposing your skin to the sunlight – your body is designed to synthesize the vitamin D it needs from it. Where it gets tricky is just how long you should expose your skin to sunlight.

Dr John Cannel, one of the leading experts on vitamin D, recommends exposing your skin to the sun just until your skin is about to turn pink. The best time to do this is near midday, when the most amount of UVB is coming from the sun. This will give you 25,000UI of vitamin D per day, which is more than enough to correct a deficiency.

However, it is not always possible to get adequate skin exposure to sunlight. In the case of winter, or if you live far away from the equator, it becomes harder for UVB to penetrate the earth's atmosphere. Therefore, Dr. John Cannel recommends that adults take a 5,000UI supplement of vitamin D Daily to correct a deficiency.

If you think you may be vitamin D deficient, speak to your doctor about getting your vitamin D levels checked. If they are low, you stand to make big gains in symptom reduction by correcting a deficiency.

Ginger

Ginger is a flowering plant in the family Zingiberaceae whose root is used as a spice and for its therapeutic qualities in Ayurvedic medicine as a natural anti-inflammatory food. Several studies have demonstrated ginger's ability to treat arthritis.

In one study, 247 participants with knee osteoarthritis were given either 255 mg of ginger capsules or placebo capsules twice a day for six months [9]. Significant reduction in knee pain was reported by 63% of the participants who were treated with ginger. The ginger group also had a reduction

in the severity of pain and overall improvement of osteoarthritis-related symptoms compared to the placebo group.

Ginger works so well because it contains compounds that act as cox-2 inhibitors. By inhibiting cox-2, less inflammatory prostaglandins are produced and therefore less pain and joint swelling.

Ginger can be obtained by using it in cooking or as a supplement in powdered form from capsules.

Curcumin

Curcumin is the active ingredient of turmeric which is a member of the ginger family. Curcumin gives turmeric it its yellow colour and is a potent anti-inflammatory. Like ginger, curcumin inhibits the cox-2 enzyme, blocking the production of inflammatory prostaglandins and therefore reducing pain.

The evidence for curcumin comes from a study in 2012 that found curcumin's ability to reduce disease activity and swelling joints in rheumatoid arthritis was significantly better than that of diclofenac sodium (voltaren) [10].

While you can get curcumin from using turmeric in cooking, taking a supplement is often more effective as the curcumin is more bioavailable. Take one 500mg capsule per day.

Gelatin

The Old Adage 'eat what ails you' may sound like out of date folklore but modern science validates what our grandmothers knew. Gelatin, made from bones and joints, can help to relieve your arthritic pain.

Gelatin contains several health promoting nutrients. One of these nutrients is, type II collagen, the major protein in joint cartilage. Type II collagen helps arthritis because it contains proteins that are required for the synthesis and repair of connective tissue throughout the body. In one study, type II collagen decreased the number of swollen joints and tender joints in rheumatoid arthritis patients [11]. A small percentage of patients actually had their rheumatoid arthritis go into remission! Another trial in patients with osteoarthritis taking type II collagen for 42 consecutive days, found an average of 26% reduction of pain in four of five patients [12]. Finally, one study found that osteoarthritis patients who took type II collagen had decreased WOMAC scores (a pain index) in 33% from baseline [13].

Gelatin can be taken in powdered form. Two tablespoons added to some fruit juice daily is enough to produce an anti-arthritic effect.

CHAPTER 5: EXERCISE

People with arthritis should be moving according to the American College of Rheumatology. People with arthritis who regularly exercise have more energy, less pain, improved sleep and better day-to-day function. Yet, fatigue from arthritis is a common reason people give for decreasing their recreational pursuits and level of physical activity.

Although it might seem counterproductive to exercise your joints when they are already painful, the workout actually helps strengthen your body and prevent further bouts of inflammation. Obviously, you can't start running or weight lifting with arthritis, but there are specific workouts that will be able to offer excellent help.

Water Workouts

Water is possibly the best exercise you can have for arthritis. The buoyancy in the water prevents excessive pressure on the joints but still manages to "exercise" them properly. Simply start swimming laps in a relaxing manner. Don't put too much effort on the movement and instead enjoy the water even as you swim through it. You can also try swimming in place or moving your hands while under the pool. It is best if the pool is warm to offer further relief to the joints.

Yoga

Yoga can involve relaxed or strenuous movement so be careful on what you enroll for. People with arthritis are advised to use a more relaxing form of yoga composed mainly of slow and long stretches as opposed to heart-pumping movements. There should also be a bit of meditation involved which may not work for arthritis but does help with blood pressure.

Walking

Relaxed walking – the kind you do when trying to enjoy the view – is the easiest form of exercise for arthritis. Choose to walk on flat terrains wearing proper shoes to prevent stressing your body. Walk only according to your body's capacity whether it's just for 10 minutes or for one hour. Walking helps strengthen the muscles and increase blood flow for proper distribution of nutrients in the body. The exercise also helps burn full-body fat which means that there will be less weight pushing on the joints.

Dance Classes

It's fun and beneficial to the body, allowing you to stay on your feet without actually noticing the strain. Of course, you're not expected to perform any complicated dance moves. Ballroom dancing is usually the way to go since it is slow and graceful, letting you move to the music in no-hurry. Much like with walking, it's best to wear something light and comfortable during these times, especially when it comes to shoes.

Strength And Resistance Training

If you have a gym at your disposal, strength training can also do wonders for arthritis. Focus on using resistance bands and isometric exercises for your joint inflammation. If you're not too sure how to proceed in the gym, having a physical therapist or personal trainer with you is usually best.

CONCLUSION

As you've seen in this book, arthritis is not a disease you can't do anything about. By modulating your diet you can take control of the disease and your life.

By eating a low fat diet, avoiding high fat animal products and nuts, you are decreasing pain by consuming less arachidonic acid that leads to the production of inflammatory prostaglandins.

By beginning on a 14-day rotation diet you are speeding up healing by eliminating any food intolerances specific to you that cause immune attacks that inflame your joints.

By loading up on natural COX-2 inhibitors, olive oil, curcumin, and ginger Inflammation can be cooled even further, mimicking how NSAIDs work.

By correcting a vitamin D deficiency with sunshine or supplements, you are calming the immune system to prevent auto-immune attacks.

By taking two tablespoons of gelatin per day you are providing your body with the raw building blocks for healthy joints.

So begin today and make a shift towards eating a more arthritis healthy diet. Implement the diet and supplements outlined in this book. Your joints will thank you for it.

Finally, if you enjoyed this book, please take the time to share your thoughts and post a review on Amazon. It'd be greatly appreciated!

Thank you and good luck!

REFERENCES

[1] Sköldstam L, Larsson L, Lindström FD. Effects of fasting and lactovegetarian diet on rheumatoid arthritis. Scand J Rheumatol 1979;8:249–55.

[2] Sköldstam L. Fasting and vegan diet in rheumatoid arthritis. Scand J Rheumatol 1986;15:219–23.

[3] Kjeldsen-Kragh J. Rheumatoid arthritis treated with vegetarian diets. Am J Clin Nutr 1999 Sep;70:594S-600S.

[4] McDougall J, Bruce B, Spiller G, Westerdahl J, McDougall M. Effects of a very low-fat, vegan diet in subjects with rheumatoid arthritis. J Altern Complement Med. 2002 Feb;8(1):71-5.

[5] Clinton C, O'Brien S, Law J, Renier C, Wendt M. Whole-Foods, Plant-Based Diet Alleviates the Symptoms of Osteoarthritis. Arthritis, vol. 2015, Article ID 708152, 9 pages, 2015.

[6] Sköldstam L, Hagfors L, Johansson G. An experimental study of a Mediterranean diet intervention for patients with rheumatoid arthritis. Ann Rheum Dis. 2003 Mar;62(3):208-14.

[7] Lucas CP, Power L. Dietary fat aggravates active rheumatoid arthritis. Clin Res 1981;29:754A

[8] Abuzakouk M, O'Farrelly C. Diet, fasting and rheumatoid arthritis. Lancet 1992;339:68.

[9] Wigler I, Grotto I, Caspi D, Yaron M. The effects of Zintona EC (a ginger extract) on symptomatic gonarthritis. Osteoarthritis Cartilage 2003; 11(11):783–9.

[10] Chandran B, Goel A. A randomized, pilot study to assess the efficacy and safety of curcumin in patients with active rheumatoid arthritis. Phytother Res. 2012 Nov;26(11):1719-25.

[11] Trentham DE, Dynesius-Trentham RA, Orav EJ, Combitchi D, Lorenzo C, Sewell KL. Effects of oral administration of type II collagen on rheumatoid arthritis. Science. 1993 Sep 24;261(5129):1727-30.

[12] Bagchi D, Misner B, Bagchi M, Kothari SC, Downs BW, Fafard RD, Preuss HG. Effects of orally administered undenatured type II collagen against arthritic inflammatory diseases: a mechanistic exploration. Int J Clin Pharmacol Res. 2002;22(3-4):101-10

[13] Crowley D, Lau CF, Sharma P, Evans M, Guthrie N, Bagchi M. Safety and efficacy of undenatured type II collagen in the treatment of osteoarthritis of the knee: a clinical trial. Int J Med Sci 2009; 6(6):312-321.

Printed in Great Britain
by Amazon

62533556R00017